Praise for *My Anxiety Disorder Does Not Have Me!*

Anxiety is often misunderstood. This book is an excellent guide and a must for your child's continuous development.

> Dr. Monica Hardy, Teacher, Author, and a Preacher. Dr. Hardy is a versatile, multi-credentialed professional with 30+ years of combined experience in Health Information Management, Human Resource Development and Adult Education.

My Anxiety Disorder Does Not Have Me! is a wonderful book that will help children to develop self–awareness, empowerment, and greater understanding of a universal human experience.

> Dr. Anita Gadhia-Smith, Psychotherapist awarded best in Washington, DC, best-selling Author, and frequent contributer to national news on the subjects of mental health and addiction.

This book is simply AWESOME! What a great way to teach our children how to handle Anxiety and improve their social, academic and behavioral progress. This book is a must have for kids, teachers, and parents.

> Adrienne Martin, CEO, Best Boss Group, Co-Author

MY ANXIETY DISORDER DOES NOT HAVE ME!

Anxiety Disorder Explained by a Child

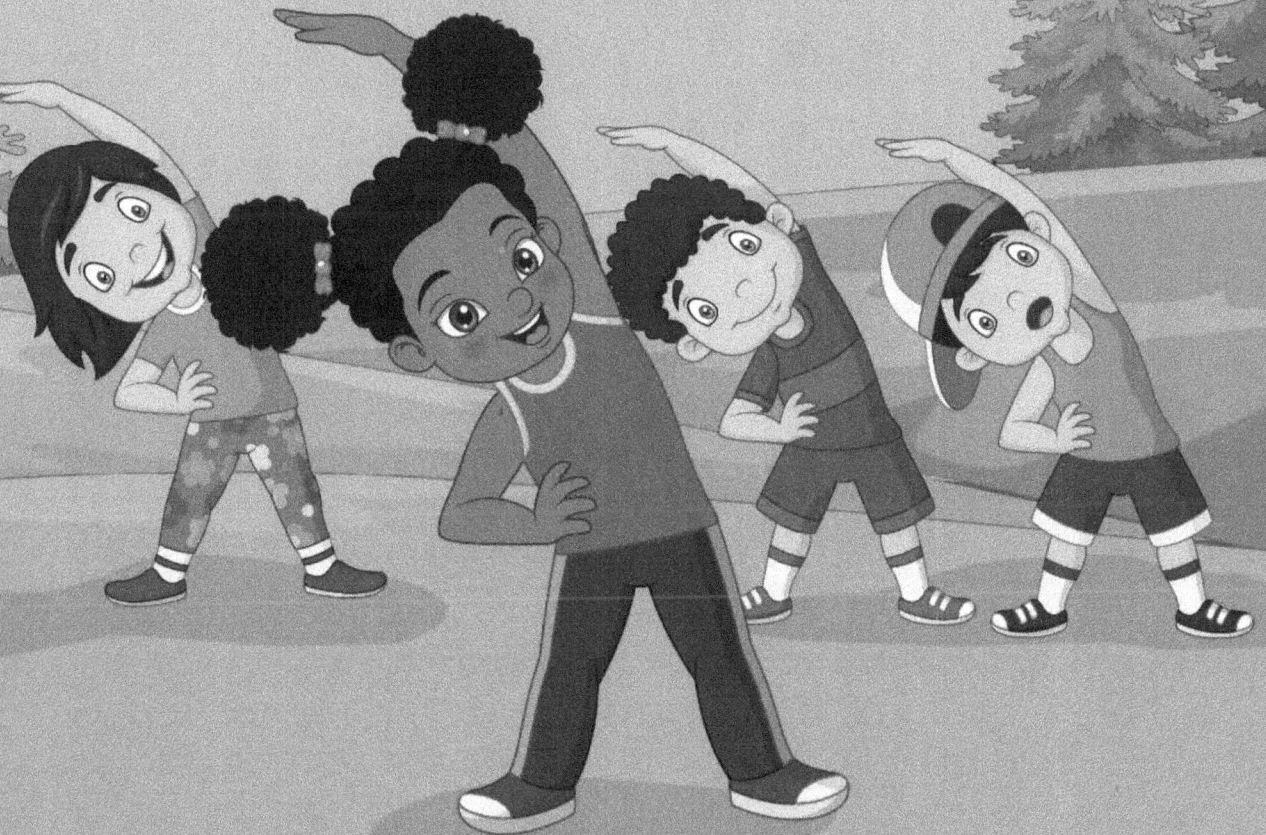

Desiree Corley Jones, LMHC

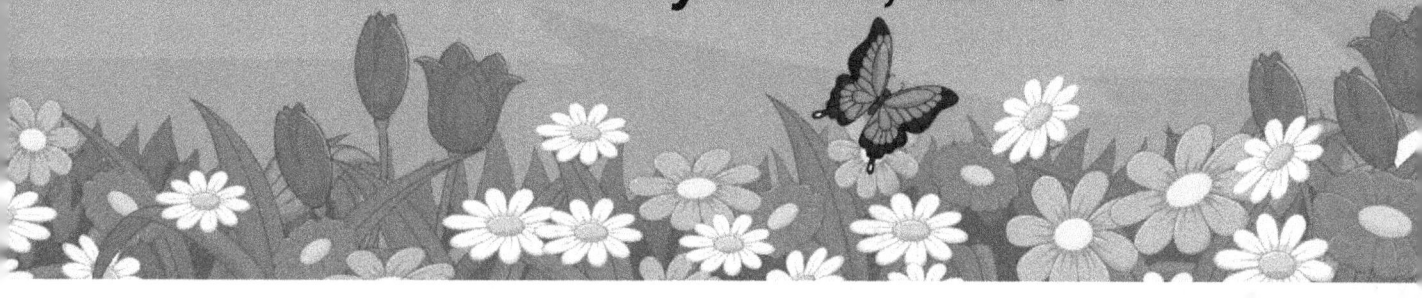

Copyright © Desiree Corley Jones
Illustrations by Attaria Zulfiqar
Edited and produced by Adrienne Hand Editing
Printed in the United States of America
All rights reserved
ISBN 979-8-218-26346-1

Published by Step-by-Step 4 Help Foundation, Inc.
Jacksonville, Florida
www.step-by-step4help.com

Dedicated to
my three children, TeJayah, Thomas, and Kevin, who
inspire me and make me so proud.
Always be the best you can be.

Mommy

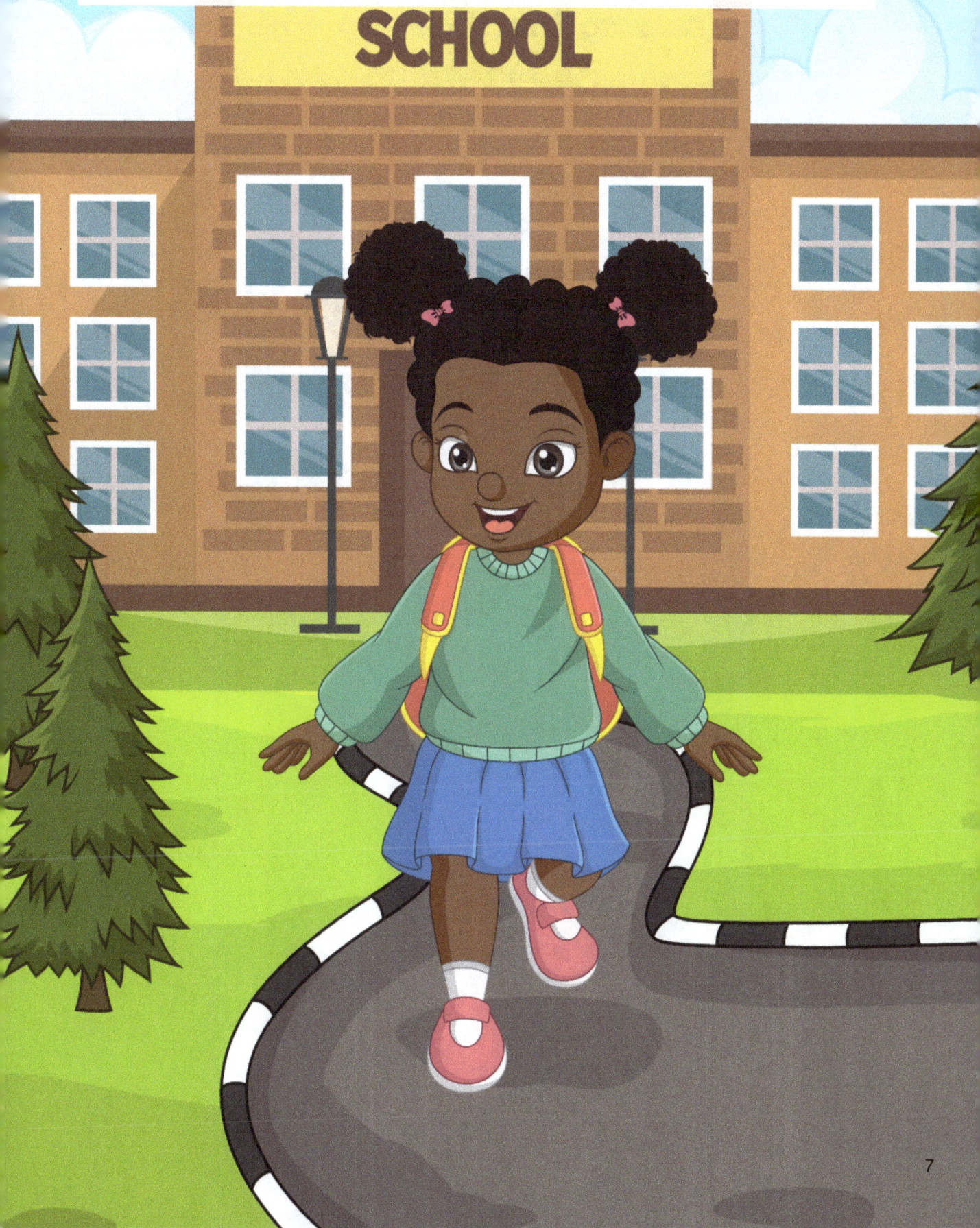

Hi, my name is Dezy! I have an Anxiety Disorder, but it does not have me!

I know what gives me butterflies now so that I can do well.

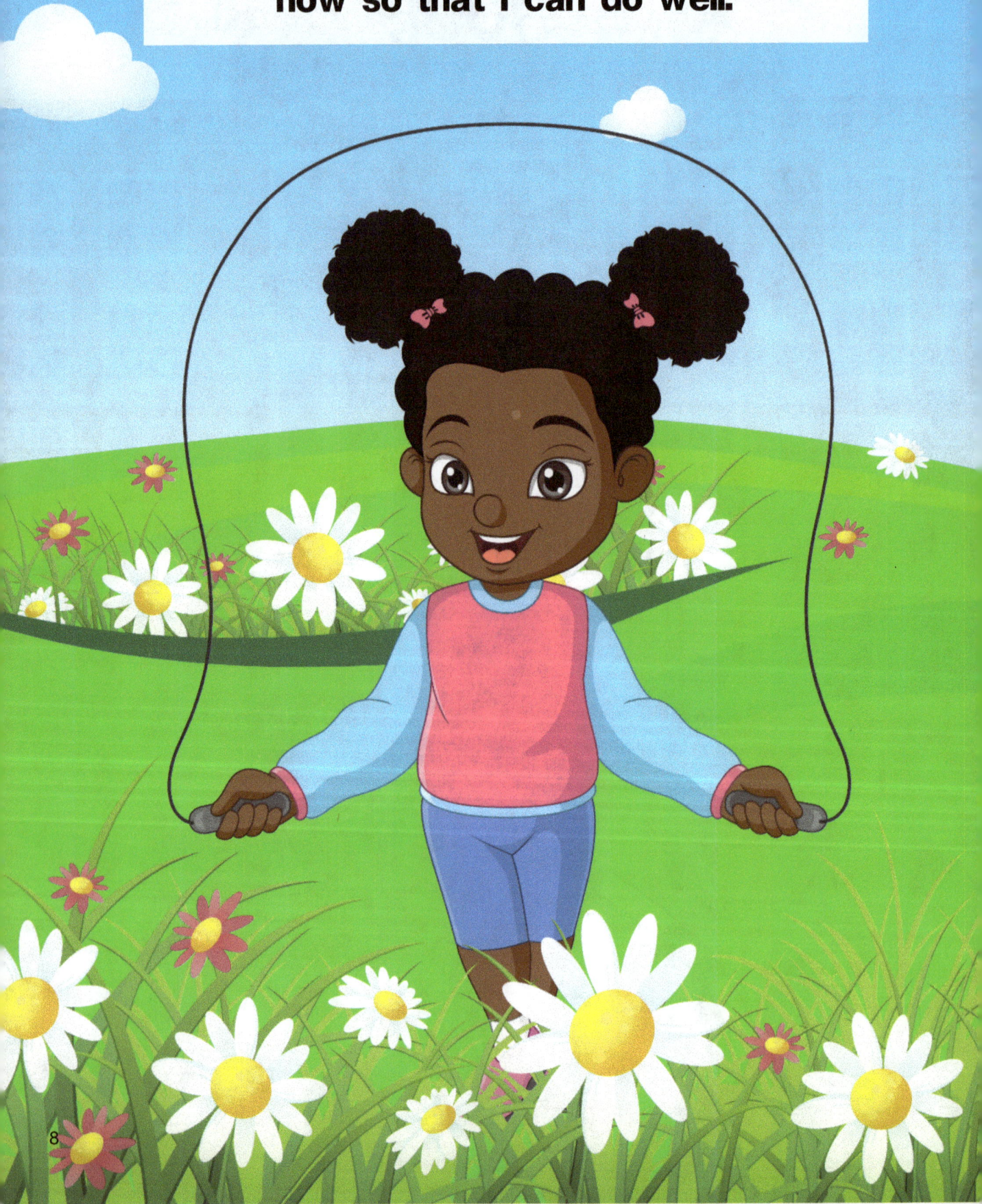

It's not that hard to tell.

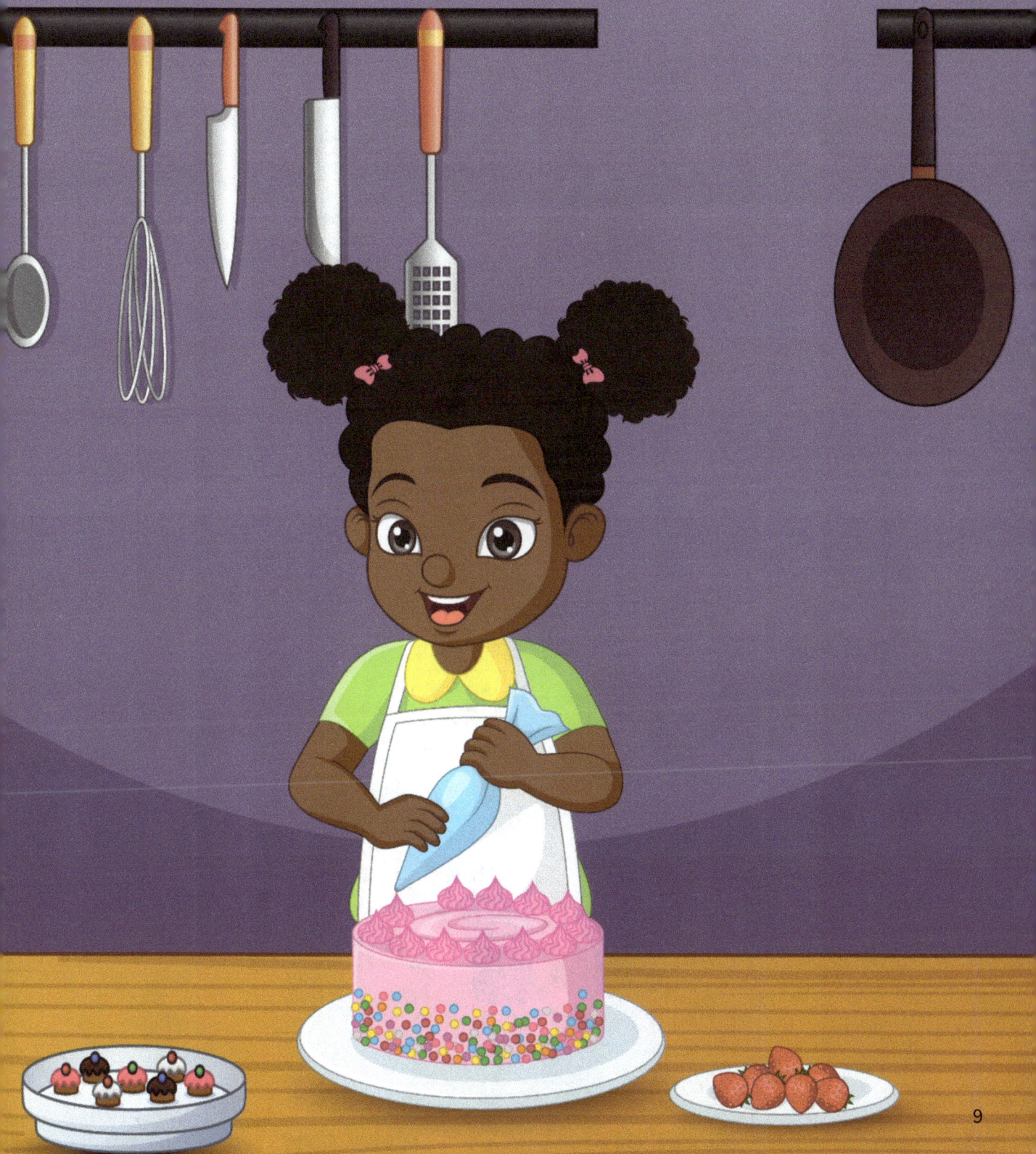

Sometimes my homework or a test
makes me feel anxious that I can't do my best.

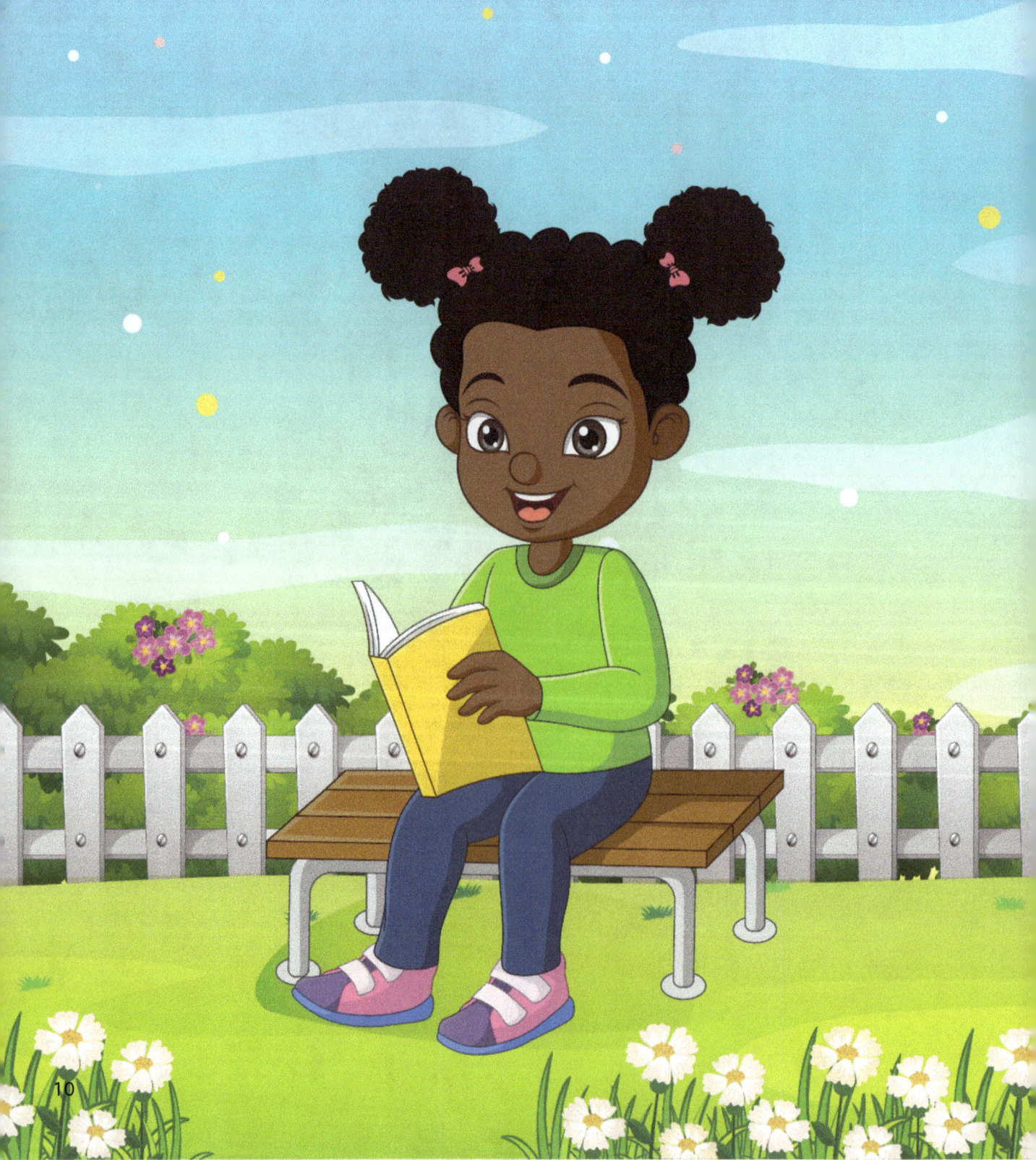

I tell my teacher how I feel,
and she gives me the help I need.

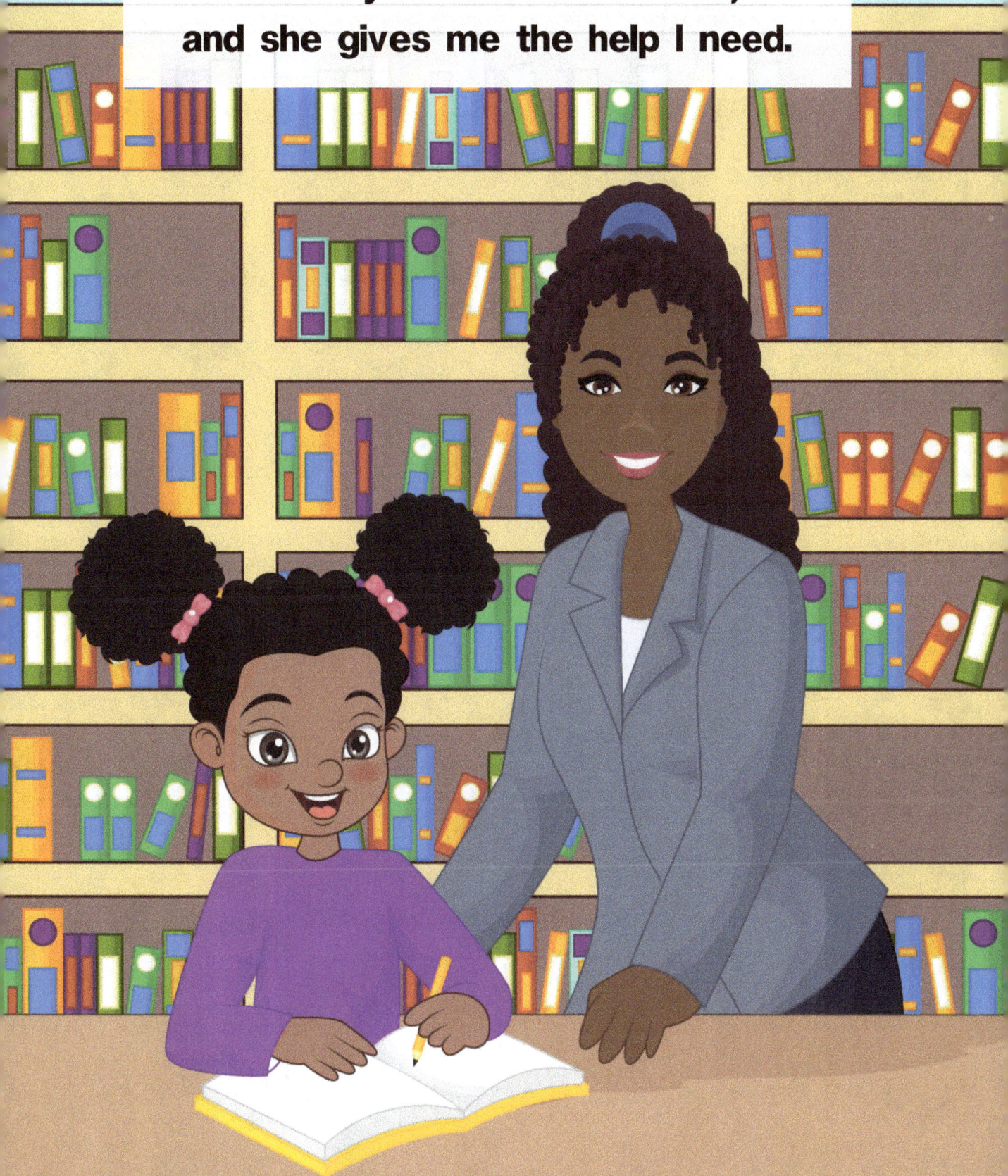

Sometimes when I make a mistake ...

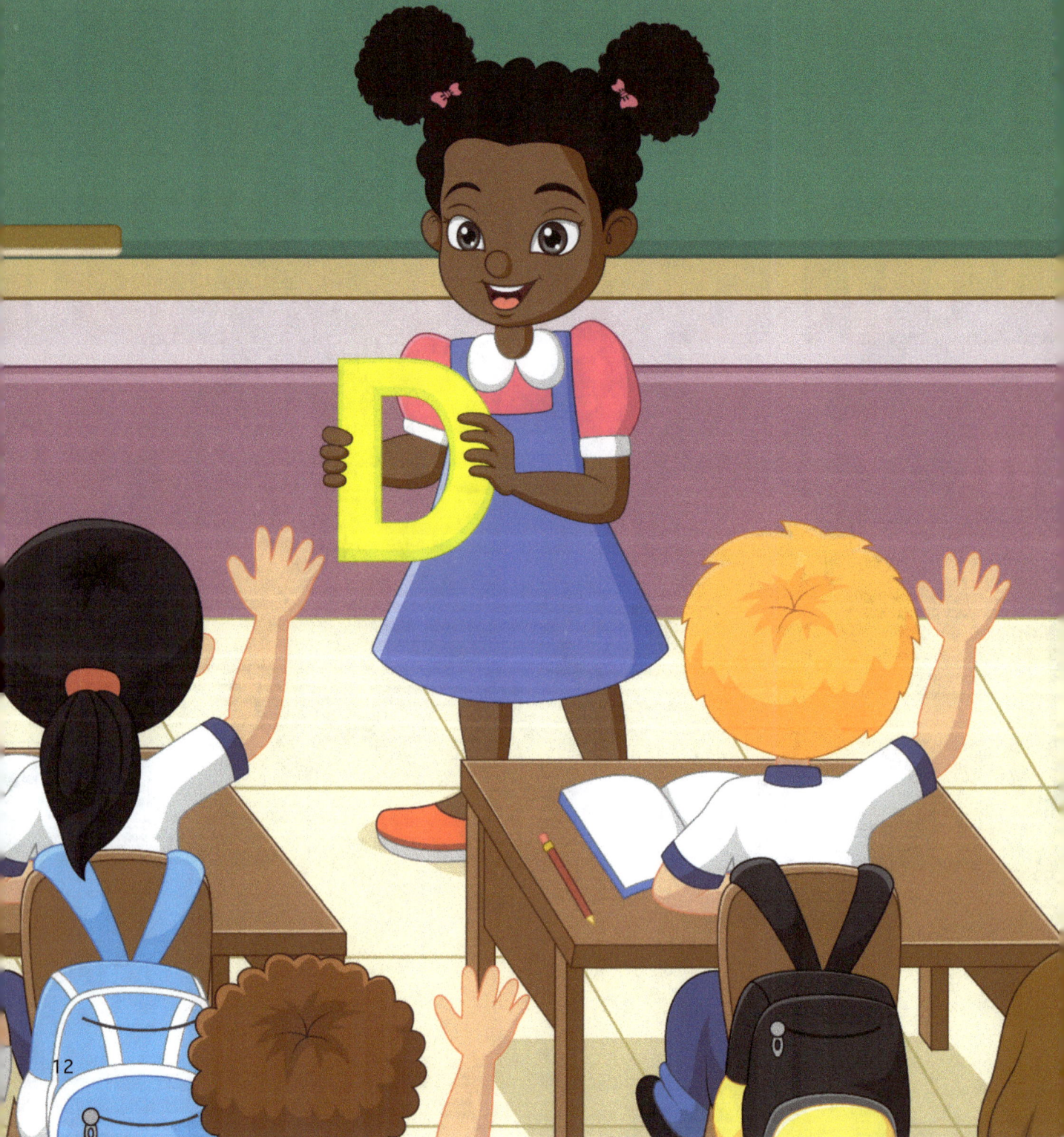

... at night, it can keep me wide awake.

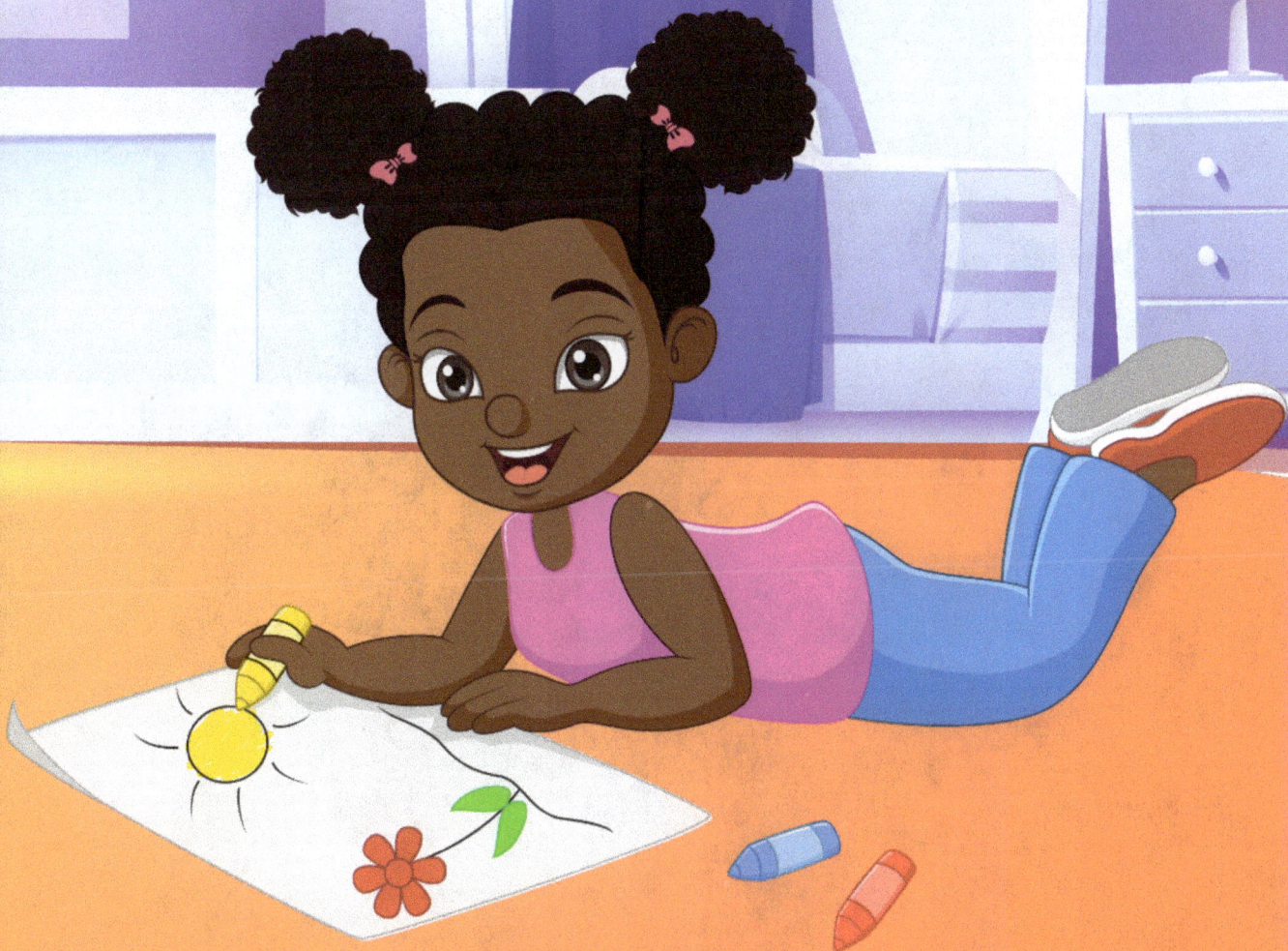

When my parents leave me all alone I cry because it's so hard to say goodbye.

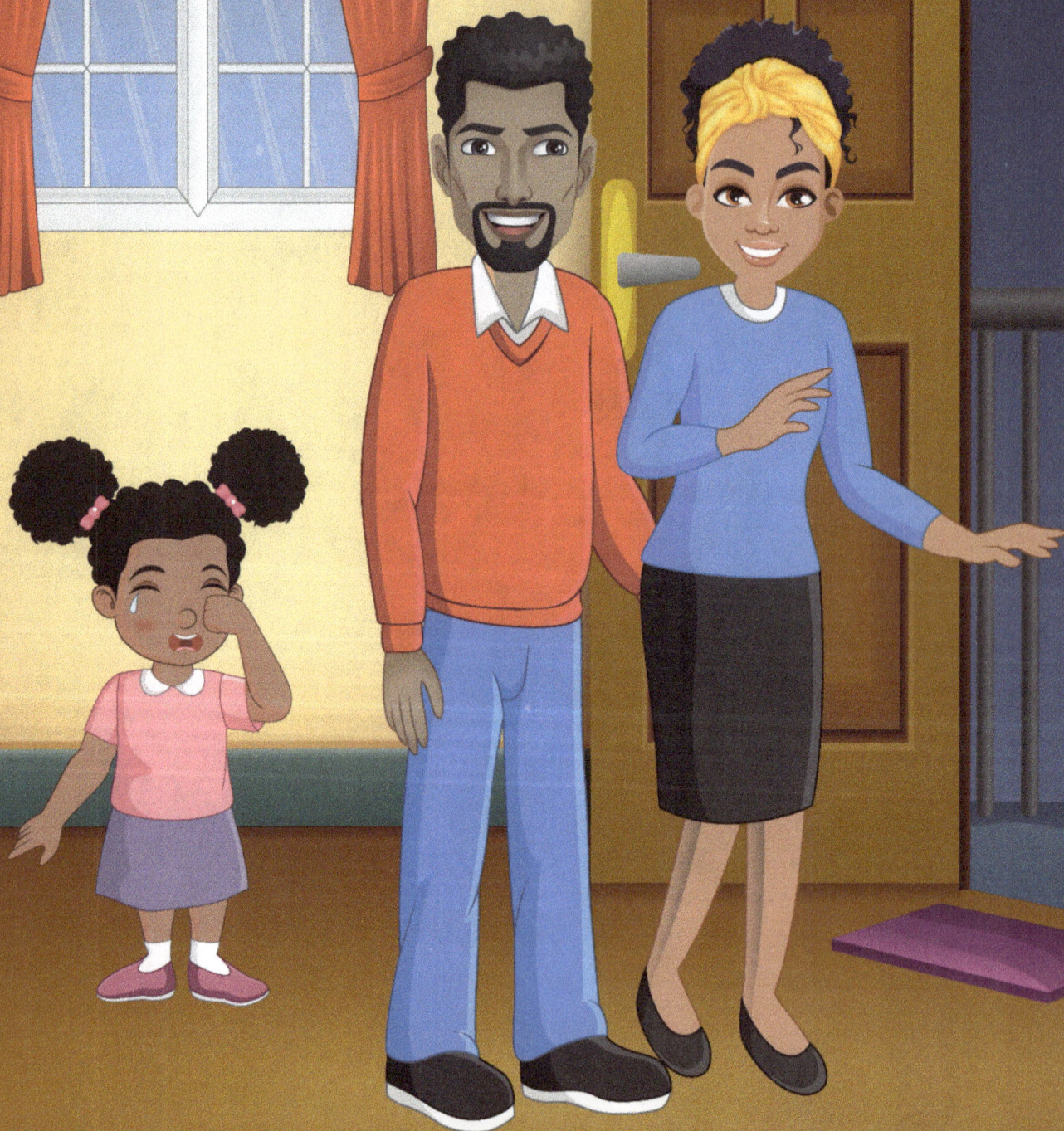

Then I change how I think and behave,
and I try to be brave.

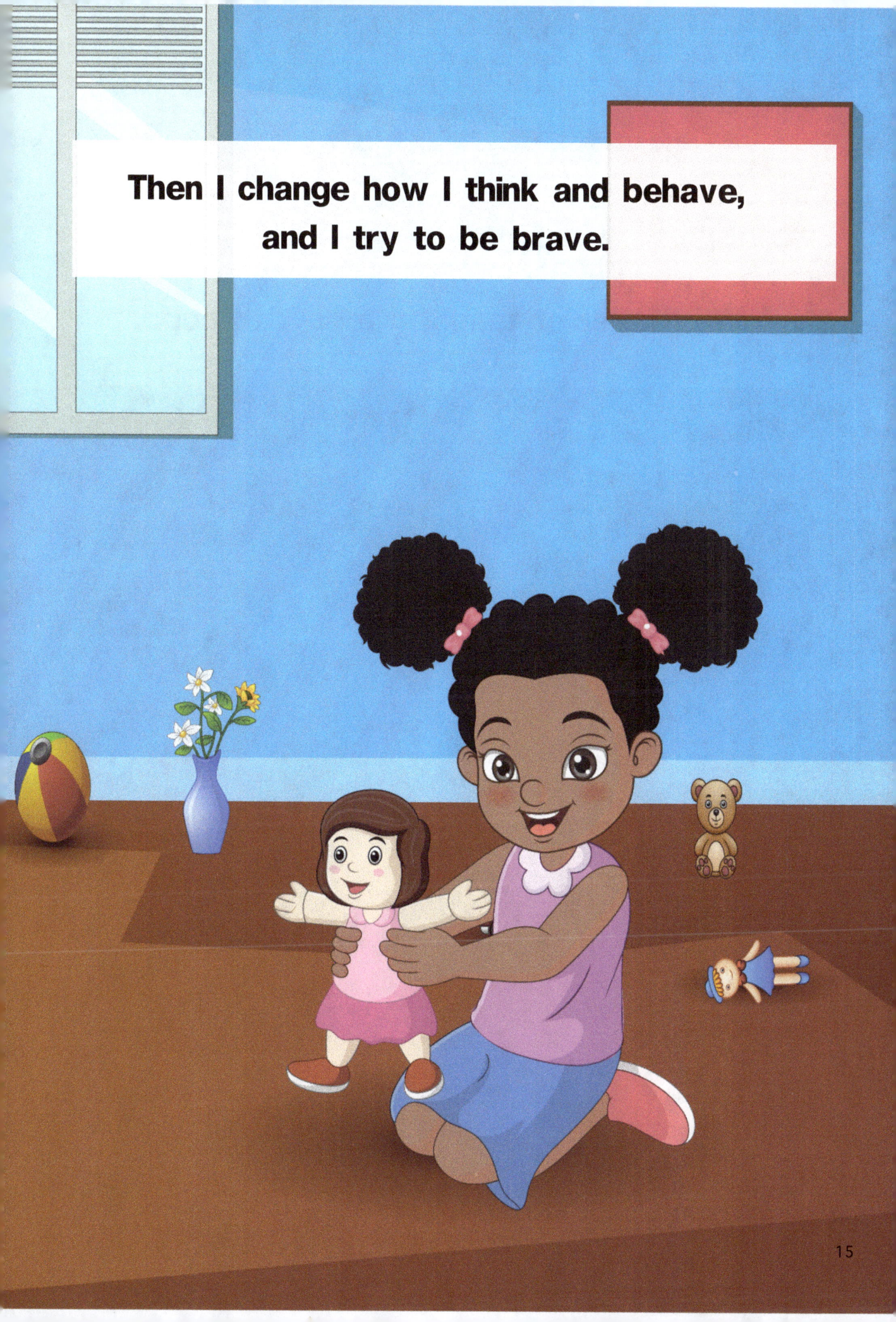

My therapist taught me how to cope.

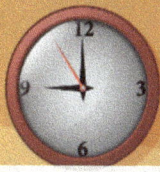

And that gives me hope!

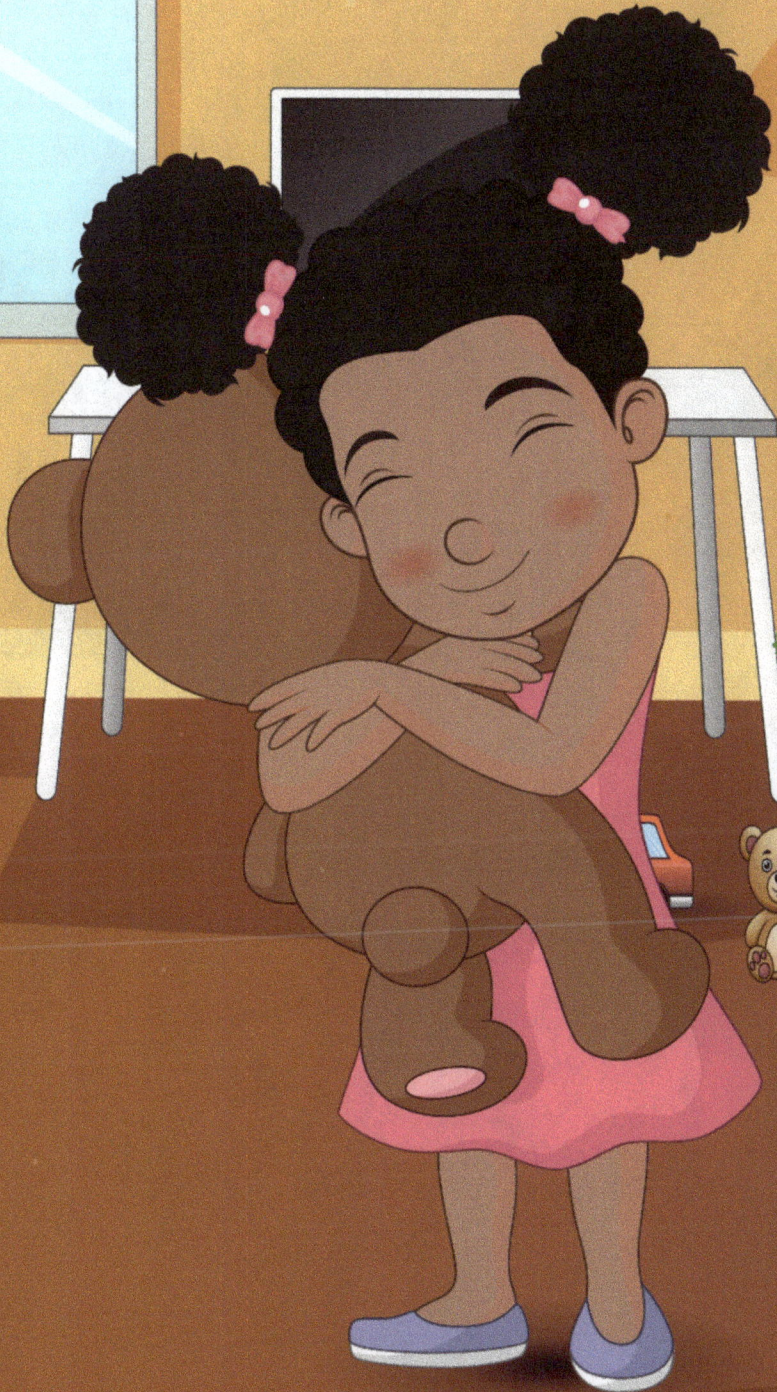

Sometimes people yell and scream because they don't know what it does to me.

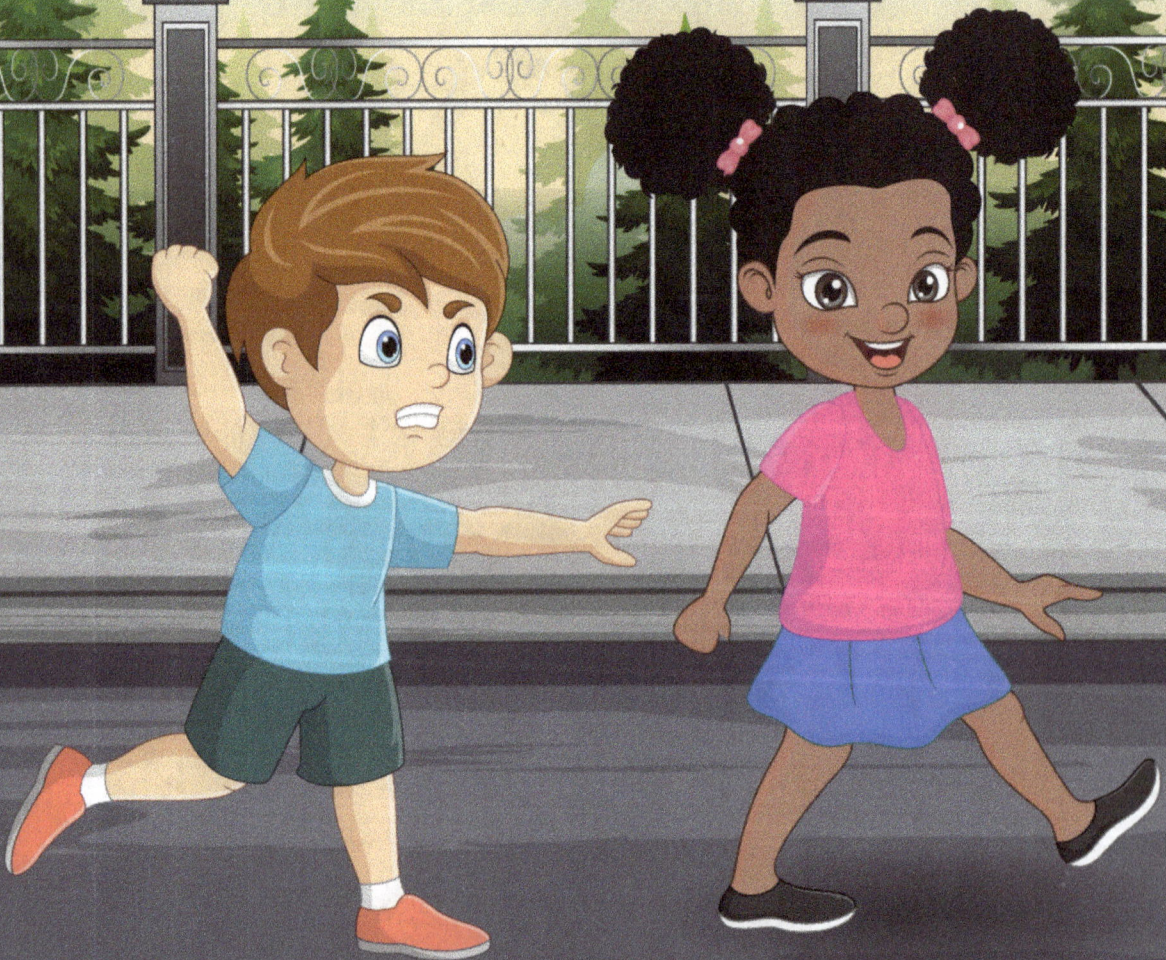

That's okay because my Anxiety Disorder does NOT have me!

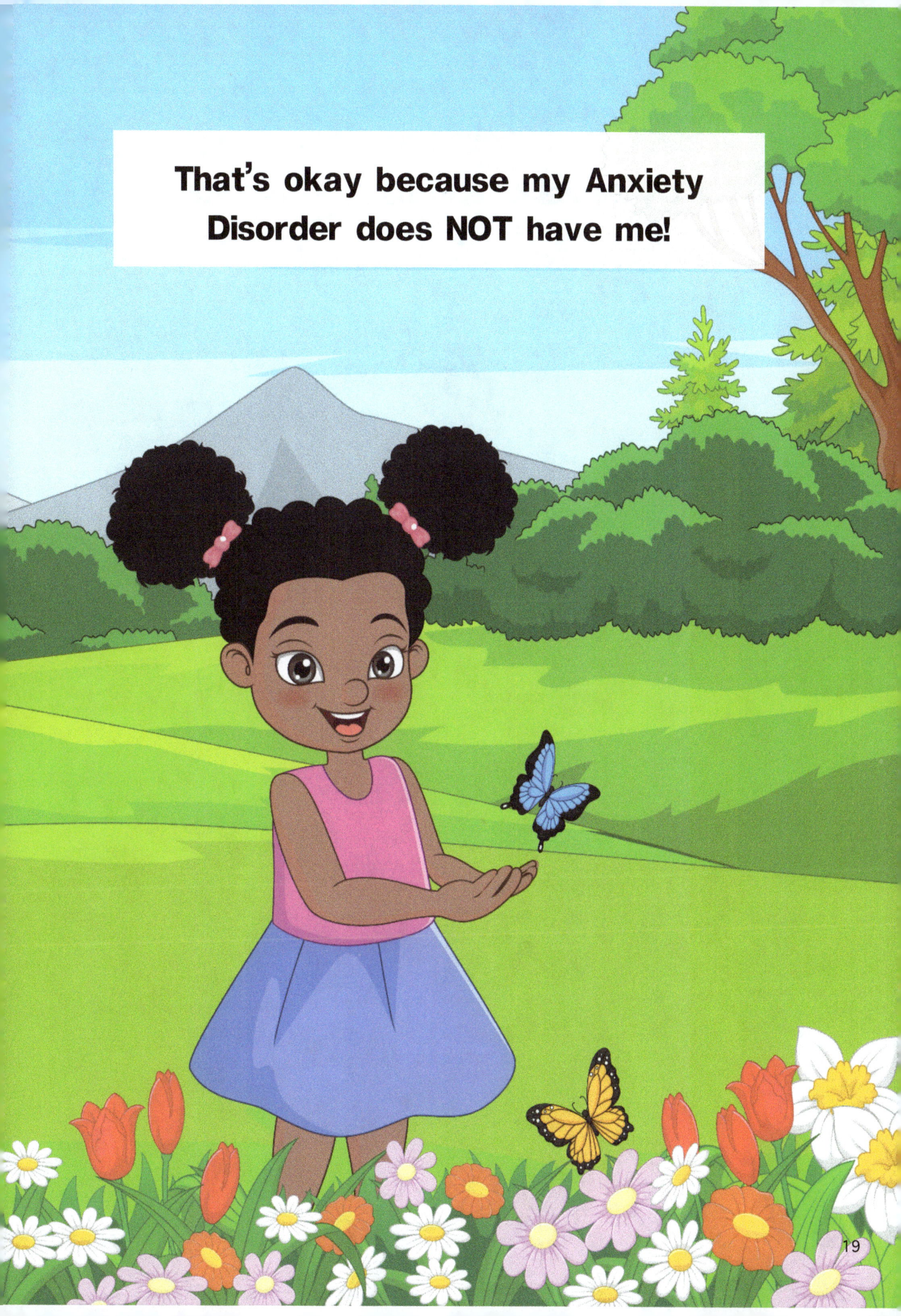

I try to relax and have some fun.

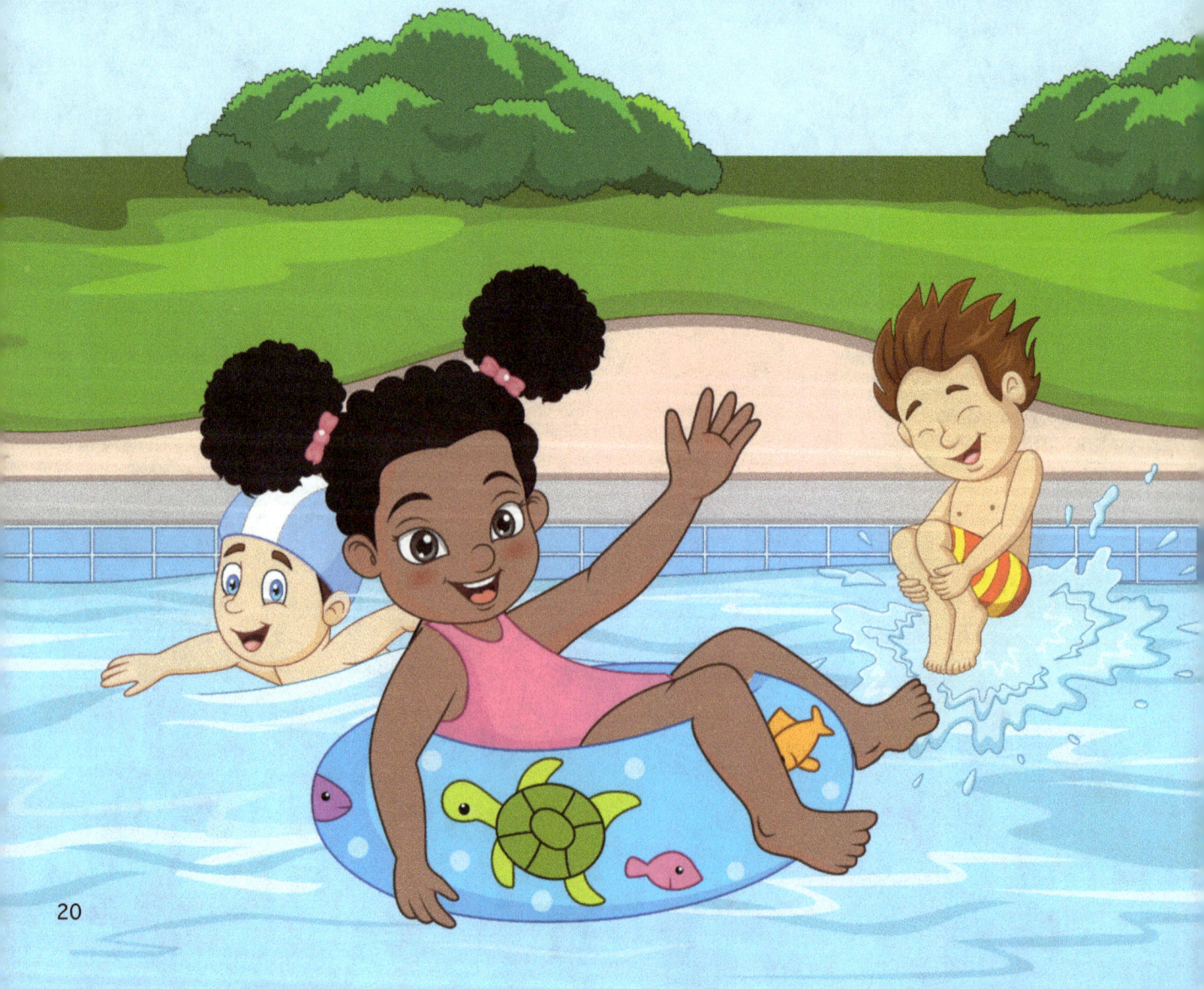

To help my mind, I go outside and take a run.

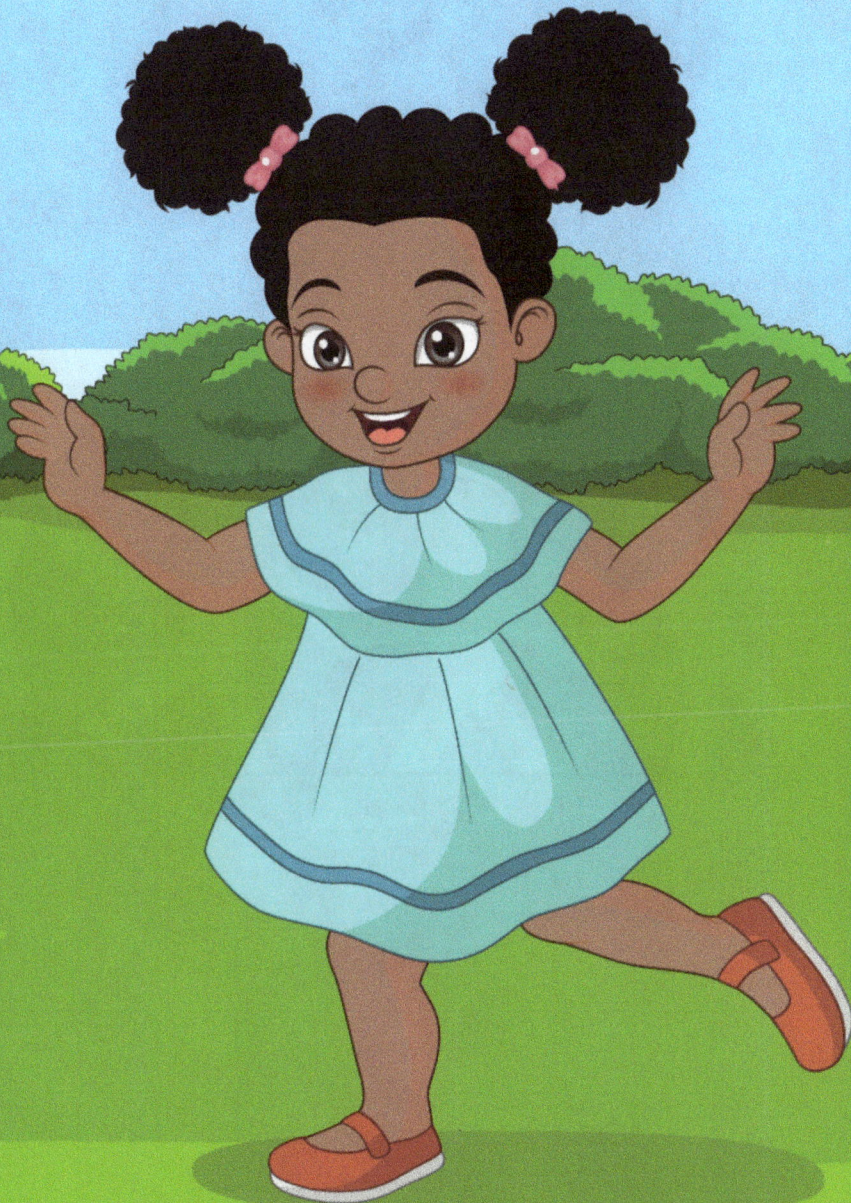

When I worry that something will happen to my family or friends ...

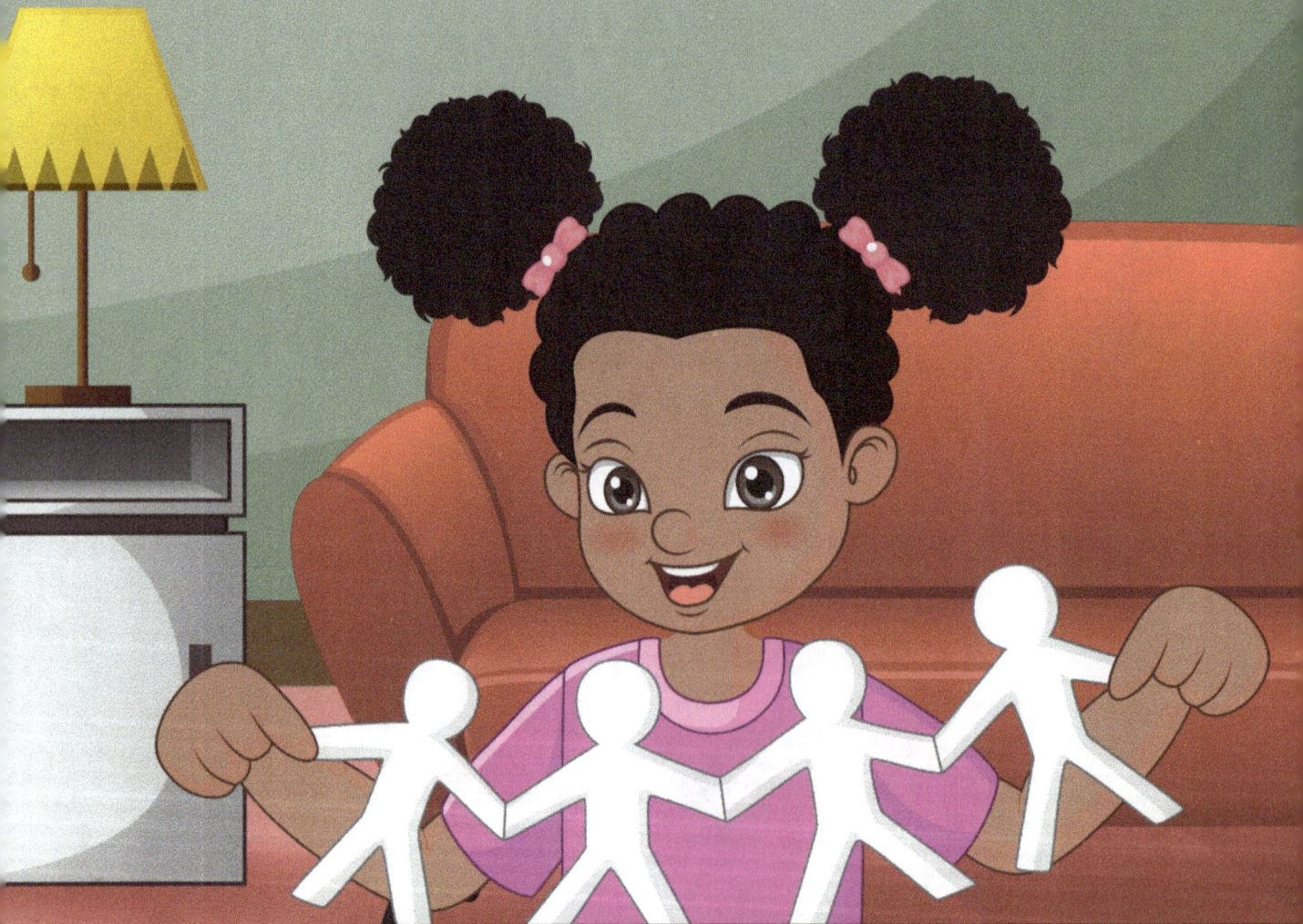

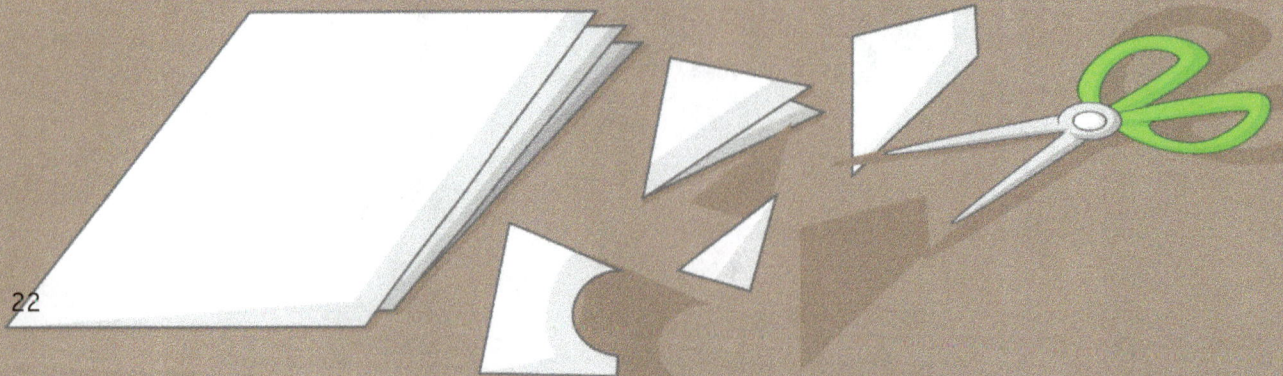

I switch my thoughts from pain and hurt
to my favorite dessert!

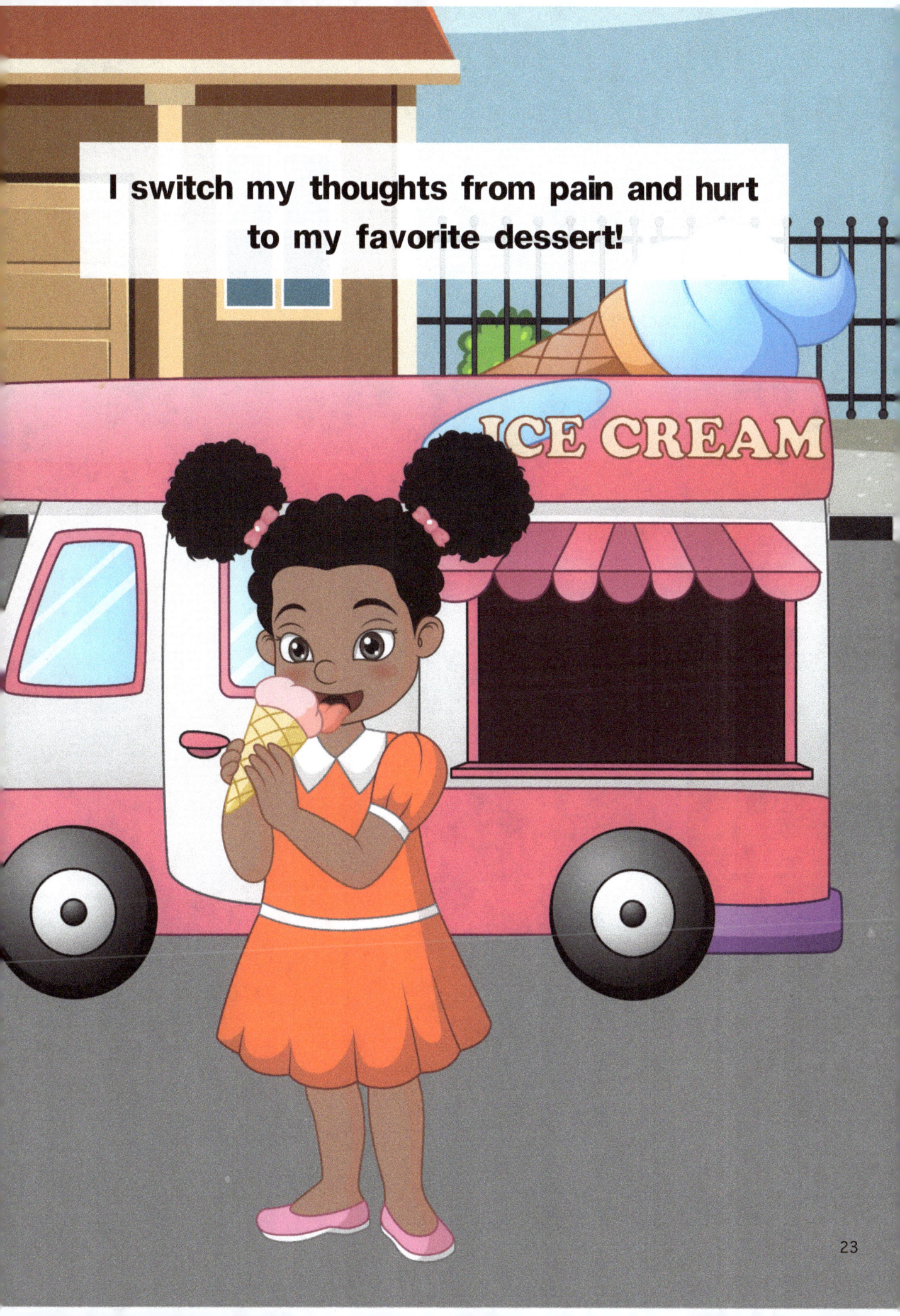

Being rude and angry is not cool.

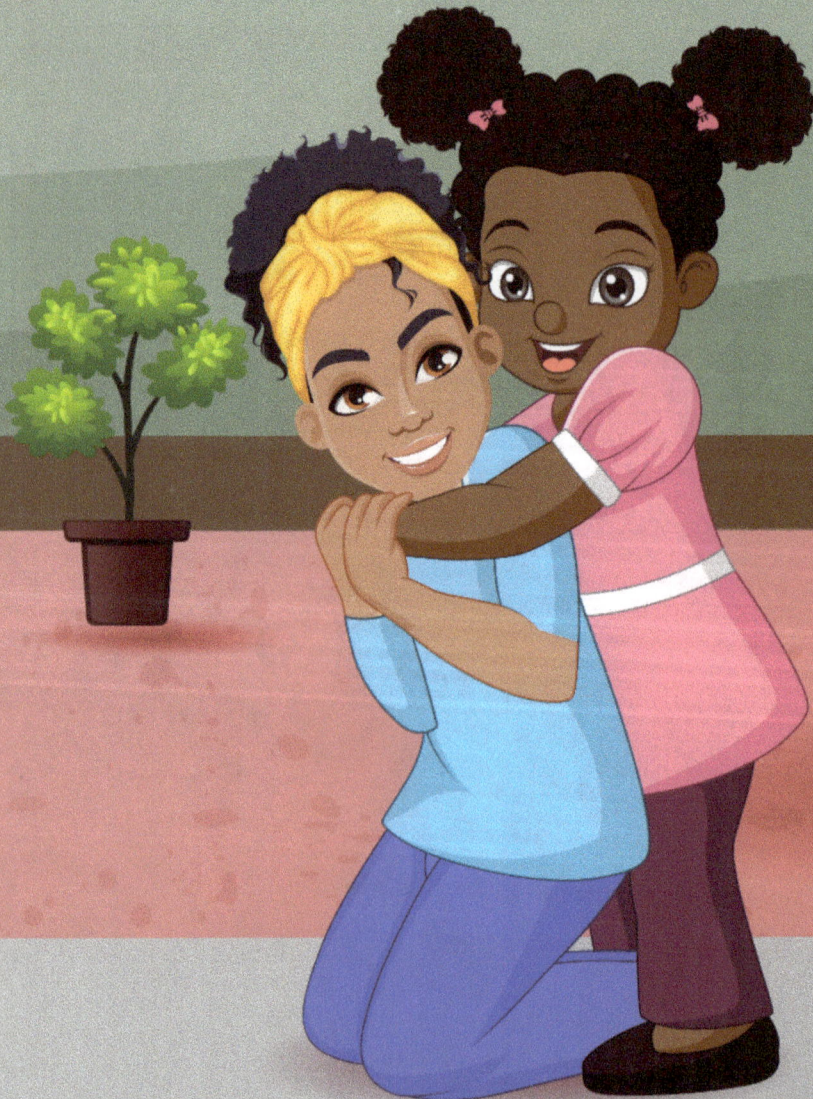

I am a smart girl who likes to do well in school.

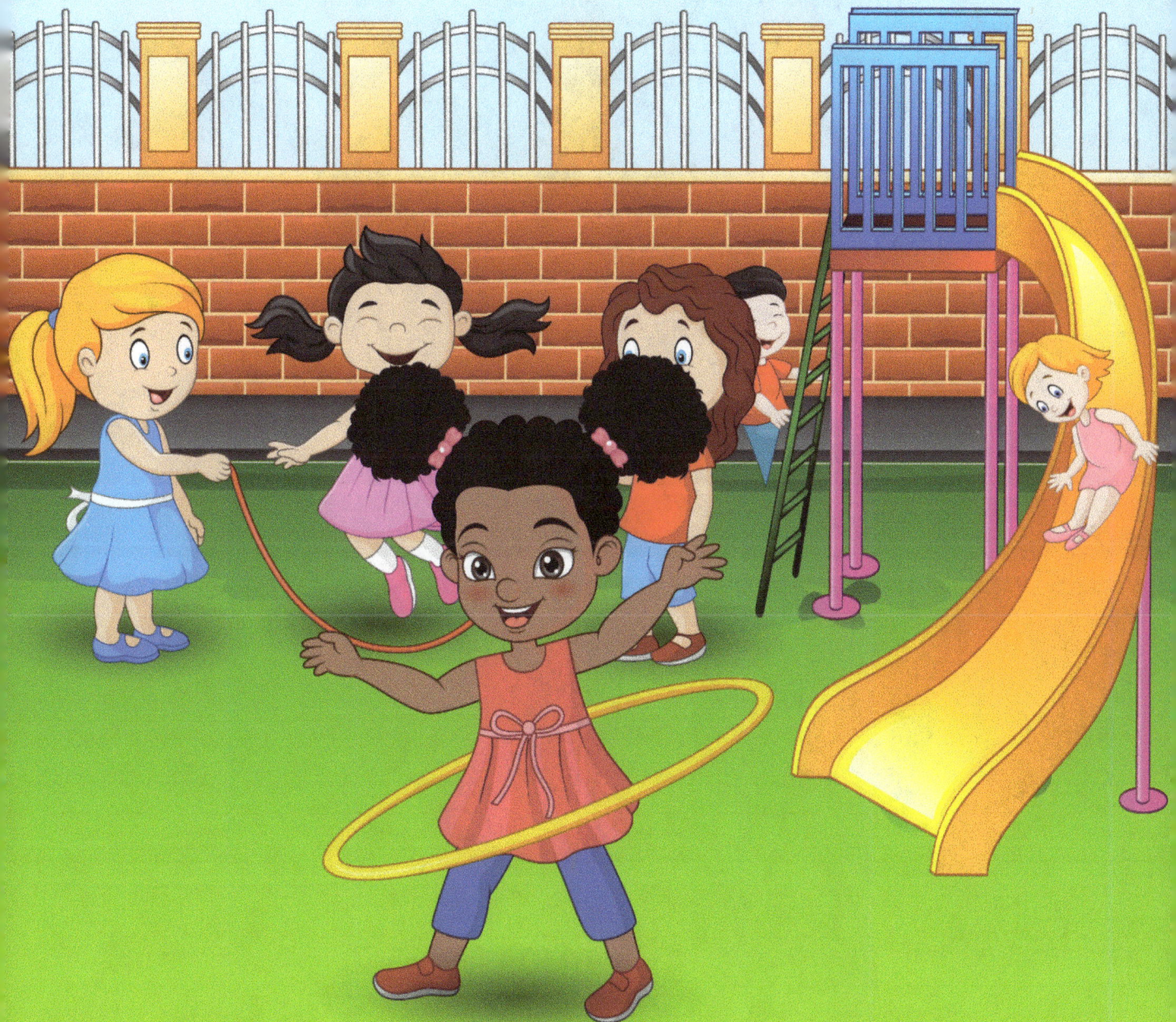

When kids laugh and are mean ...

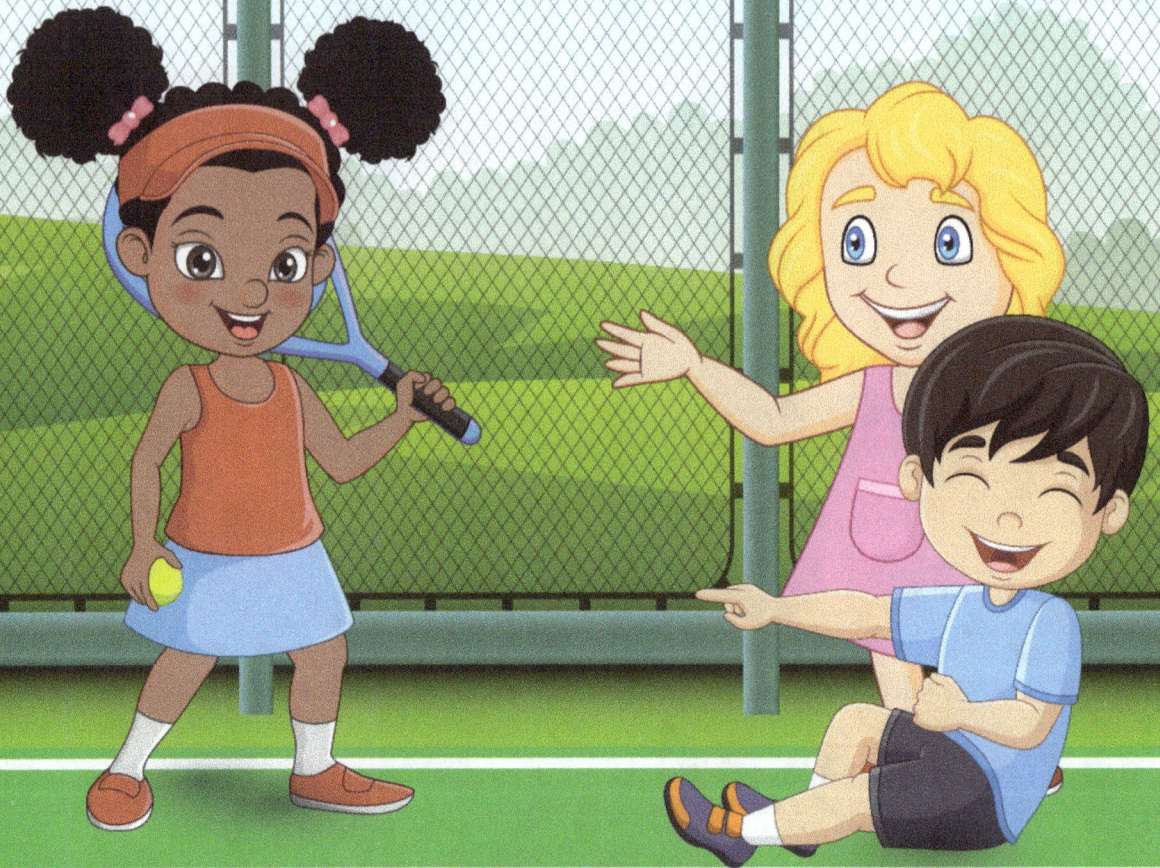

I smile because I know I am a QUEEN!

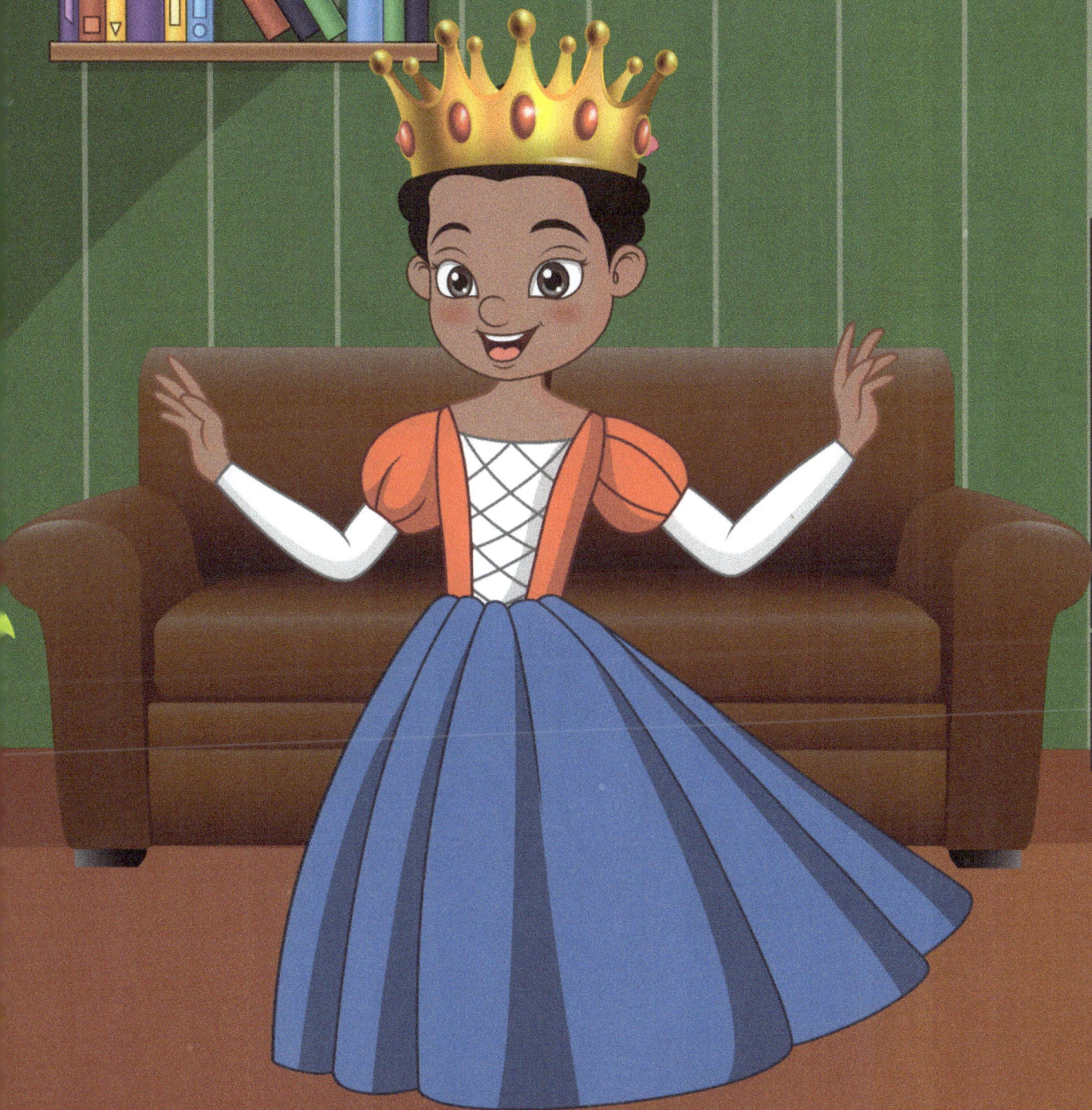

When my hands sweat and my heart beats fast, I count from 1-2-3.

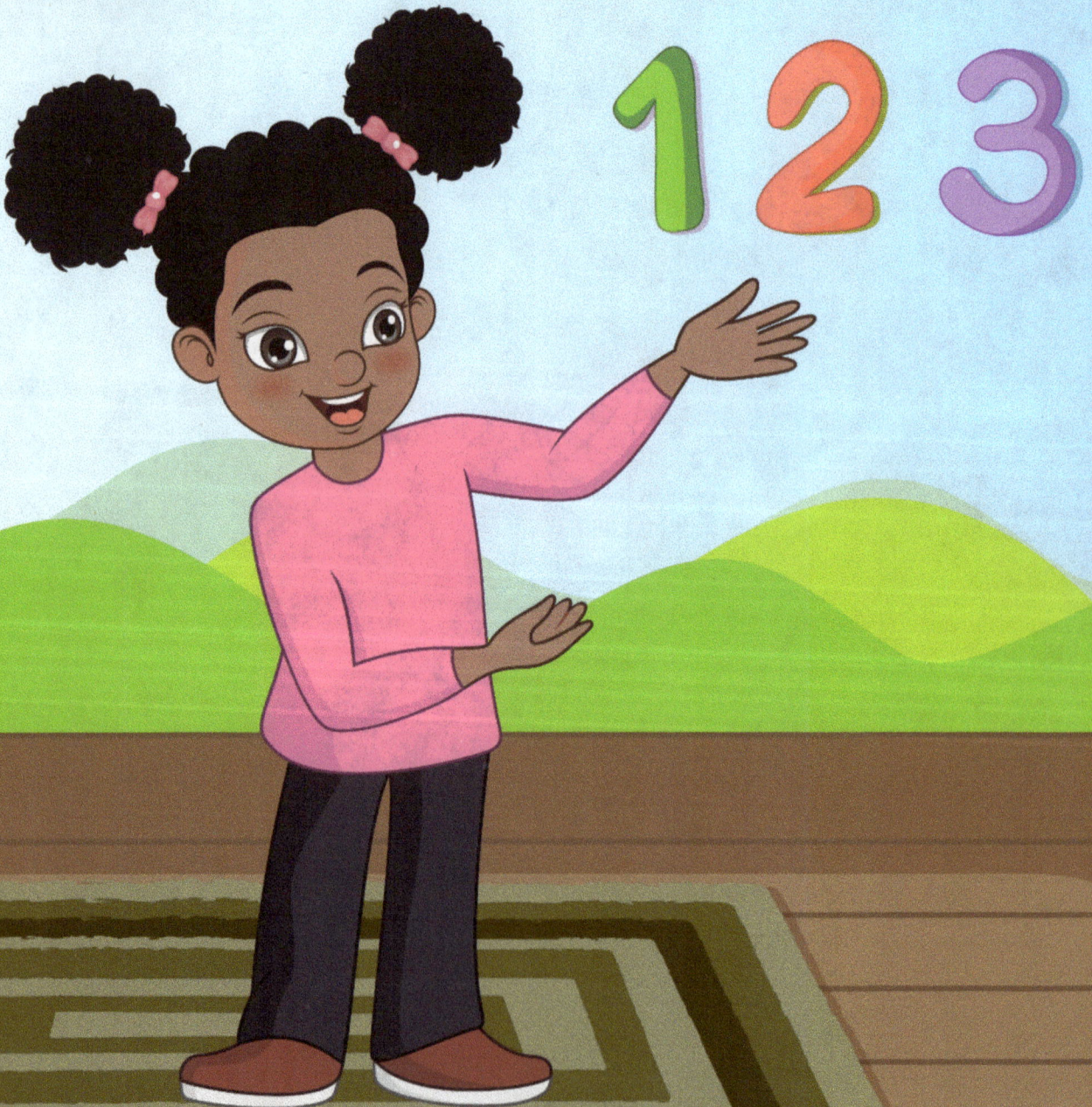

That is the Key.

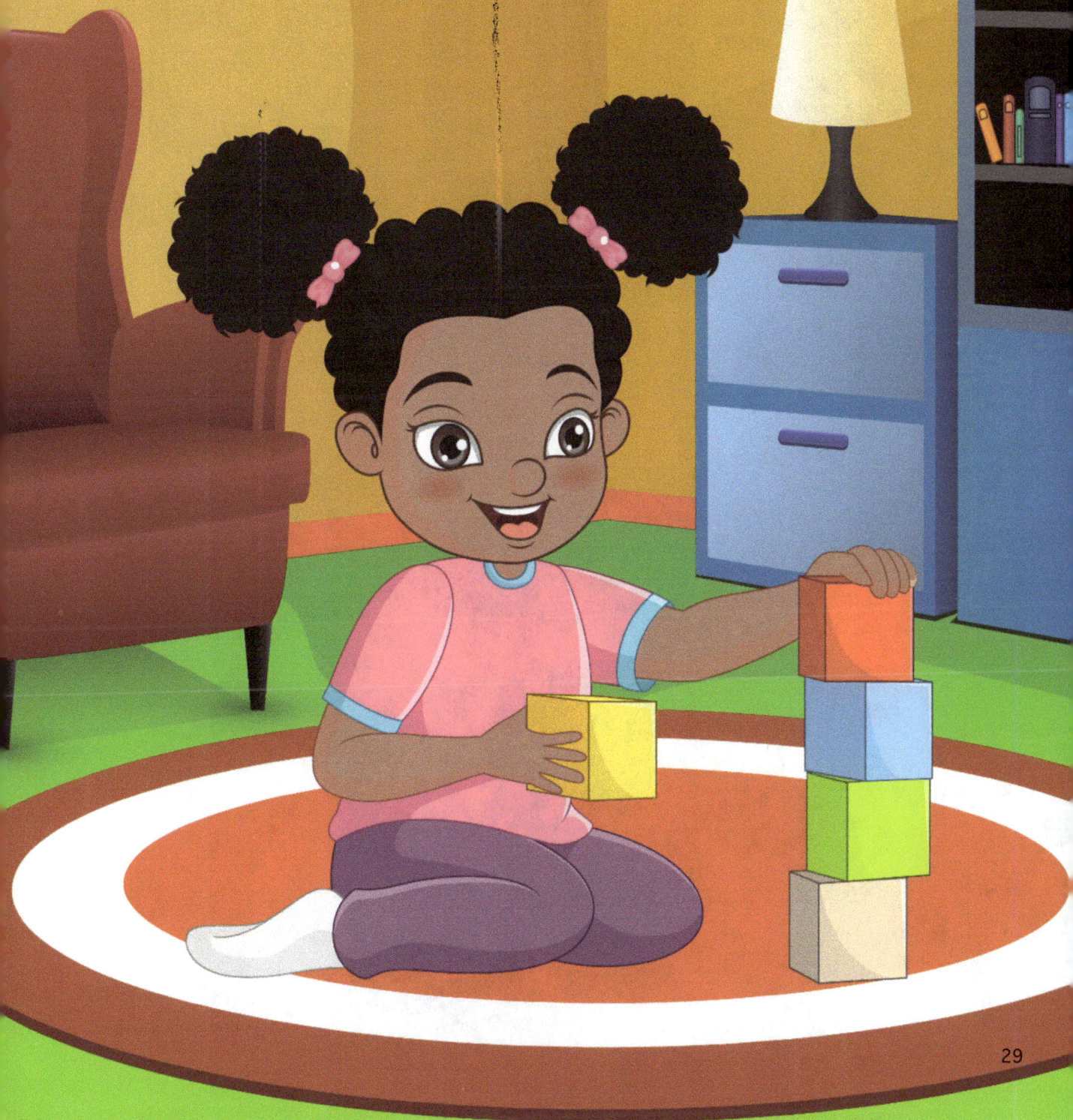

Because my Anxiety Disorder Does Not Have Me!

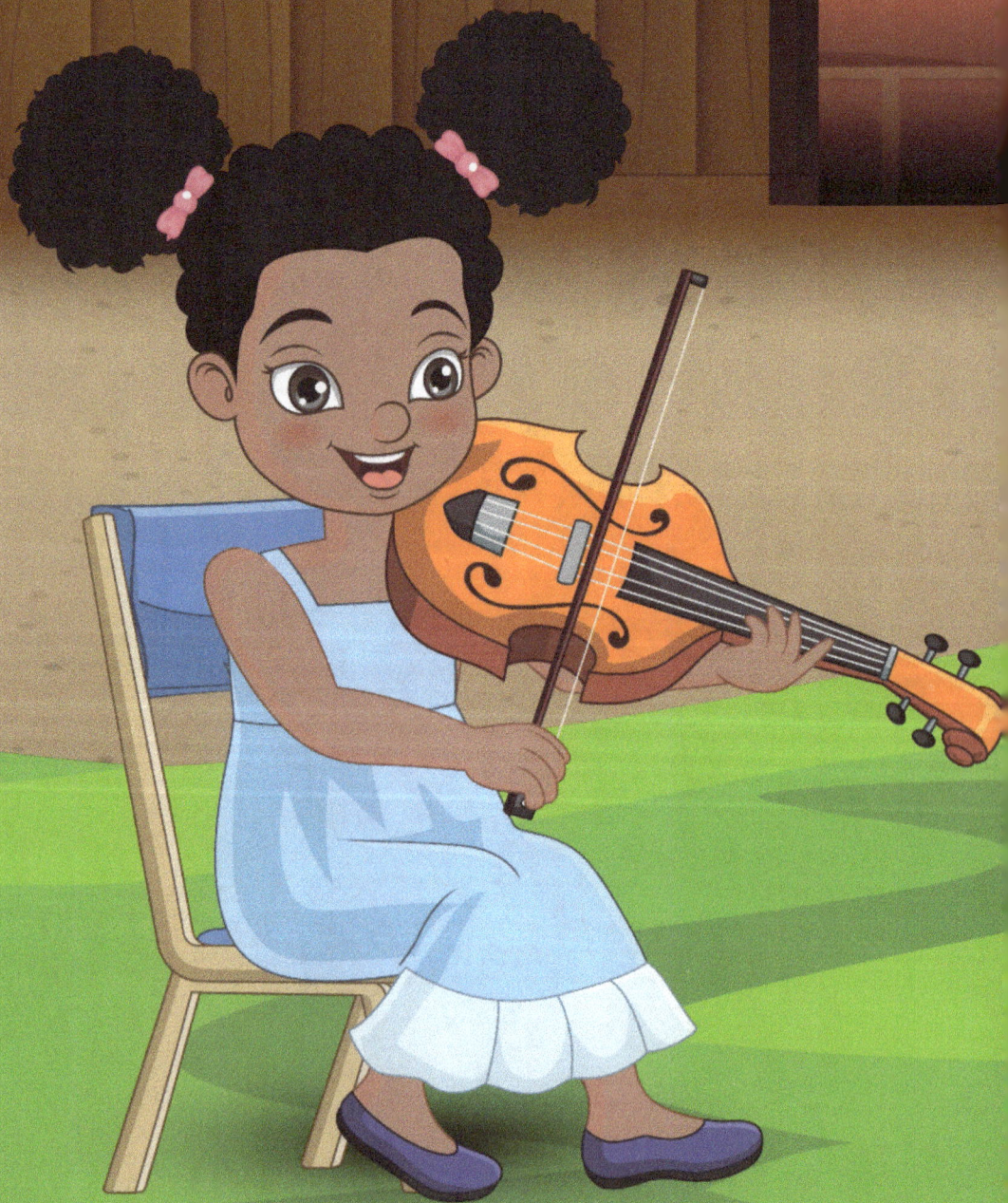

Words I Can Say Every Day

I CAN DO WHATEVER I PUT MY MIND TO

I BELIEVE IN MYSELF

I AM PERFECT JUST THE WAY I AM

I AM CREATIVE

I AM LOVED

I LOVE MYSELF

I CAN WORK WITH MY ANXIETY

I HAVE A CLEAR MIND

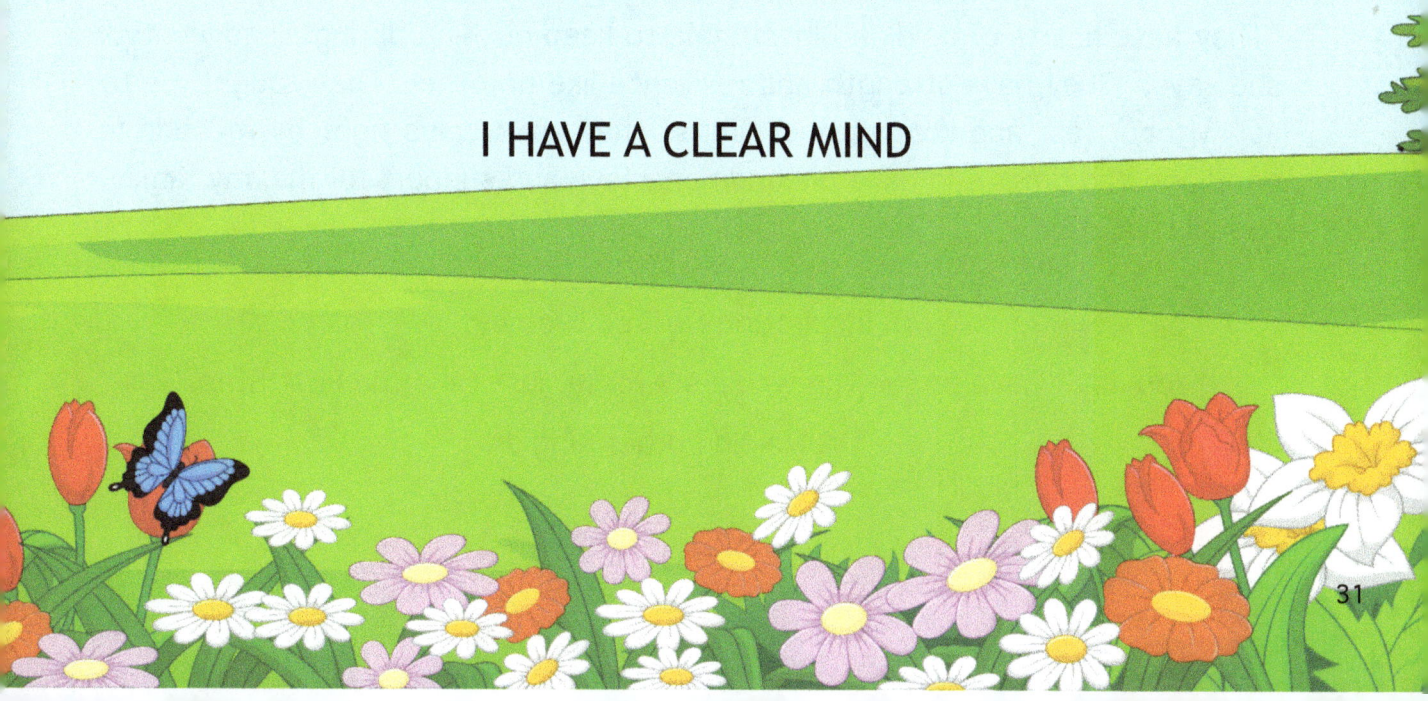

About the Author

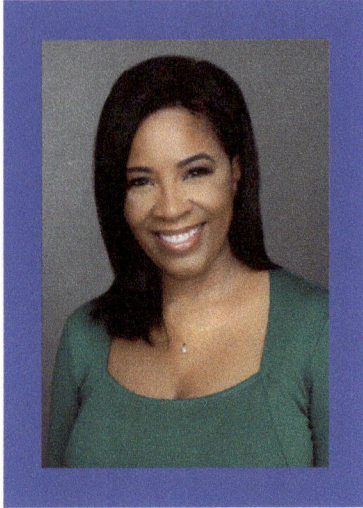

Desiree Corley Jones is the Owner and Chief Executive Officer of both Step-by-Step Behavioral Health and Step-by-Step 4 Health Foundation, Inc., as well as a licensed mental health counselor.

She lives in Jacksonville, Florida with her husband, daughter, twin boys, and their dogs.

Desiree is a proud graduate of William M. Raines High School, Bethune Cookman College, and Webster University. A member of Delta Sigma Theta Sorority, Inc., she was awarded the 2023 JAX Chamber of Commerce Small Business Leader of the Year for the Three Rivers Council. Desiree was also awarded the Best Boss Award for the Best Non-Profit and Best Healthcare Services (2021), and the News 4 JAX The One to Watch Award. In 2016, she was a Child Abuse Prevention Honoree.

Inspired by helping others realize and reach their fullest potential, Desiree strives every day to make a difference in people's lives while bringing awareness to mental health.

If you can heal from your trauma, and tap into your passion, you can "Make Your Pain Pay You!"

Her heroes and mentors include her sisters Arellia Corley and Shakesha Swift.

"They have hearts of gold and inspire me to keep pushing during all adversity," she says. "They have strength and resilience like no other. They taught me to act without fear and love without limits. They are always right by my side in good and bad times and have unconditional love and support for me, my family, and all that I do."

An inspiration Desiree lives by:

"You don't have to see the whole staircase, just take the First Step."

— Dr. Martin Luther King Jr.

Advocacy for Healthy Mental Living For All

In the US today, 1 in 5 children have a mental, emotional, or behavioral disorder, yet only 20% of these children receive care from a specialized mental health care provider. Many familes have to travel long distances or be placed on long waiting lsts to receive care. Other obstacles include affordability, lack of internet and/ or transportation, social stigma, and misinformation.

Our children deserve better.

In 2008, Desiree Corley Jones, LMHC, founded Step-by-Step 4 Help Foundation, Inc. in Jacksonvlle, Florida, and in 2016, she founded Step-By-Step Behavioral Health Services in Gainesvlle, Florida to strengthen and empower chldren, families, communities, and schools.

The mission of the Foundation is to reduce the stigma related to mental illness, intensify parental engagement, and reduce crime to create safer communities.

https://www.step-by-step4help.com

The mission of Step-by-Step Behavioral Services is to improve the lives of children and their families and to assist them in reaching their fullest potential, guiding them step-by-step. Licensed, trained counselors provide integrated, quality, compassionate mental health treatment and services that support social-emotional wellness and growth.

Step-by-Step Behavioral Services include outpatient psychiatric services, psychosocial rehabiltation, community support, individual and family therapy, therapeutic behavioral on-site therapy, and mental health training in Gainesvile and Jacksonville, Florida.

https://step-by-stepbehaviorhealth.com

"We envision a world in which all people have access to information and treatment that can help them improve their mental, behavioral, and emotional health, and achieve harmony, thus promoting healthier families, schools, and communities."

Desiree Corley Jones, LHMC

Upcoming books and workbooks
by Desiree Corley Jones, LMHC

My Bipolar Disorder Does Not Have Me!

My Depression Does Not Have Me!

My Trauma Does Not Have Me!

Anxiety and Mental Health Resources
for Teachers and Parents

Anxiety in the Classroom is an online resource center for school staff, students, and their families.

This website provides useful information, resources, and materials about anxiety and OCD as they relate to the school setting. In addition, it offers specific tools for teachers, administrators, and other school personnel who may work with students with anxiety and/or OCD. Parents/caregivers and students can also find tools and information to help them advocate for school accommodations, as well as to educate their teachers and classmates about OCD and anxiety.

https://anxietyintheclassroom.org/

Child Mind Institute
The Child Mind Institute advances children's mental health by providing evidence-based care, delivering educational resources, training educators in underserved communities, and developing breakthrough treatments.

Anxiety is the most common emotional problem in children. Kids with anxiety respond well to treatment, but it is often overlooked or misunderstood. Anxiety can show up as headaches, stomach aches, extreme shyness, and tantrums.

This website offers information and guidance for parents and teachers of children with anxiety.

https://childmind.org/topics/anxiety/

American Academy of Child and Adolescent Psychiatry
Anxiety in children is expected and normal at specific times in development. For example, from approximately age 8 months through the preschool years, healthy youngsters may show intense distress (anxiety) at times of separation from their parents or other caregivers with whom they are close. Young children may have short-lived fears, (such as fear of the dark, storms, animals, or strangers). Anxious

children are often overly tense or uptight. Some may seek a lot of reassurance, and their worries may interfere with activities. Parents should not discount a child's fears. Because anxious children may also be quiet, compliant and eager to please, their difficulties may be missed. Parents should be alert to the signs of severe anxiety so they can intervene early to prevent complications.

https://www.aacap.org/

www.ingramcontent.com/pod-product-compliance
Lightning Source LLC
Chambersburg PA
CBHW080428030426

42335CB00020B/2645